MW00415655

HELP ME ELIMINATE MY PAIN DOC!

Dr. Jerry Dreessen DC

Preface

Hello, My name is Dr. Jerry Dreessen and I'm the Owner/Treating Doctor at Back To Action Chiropractic Clinic and Massage in Mountlake Terrace, WA. In my nearly 30 years of practice, I've treated a lots people in pain, who came to me for help.

It's my mission to create a user-friendly educational system to help people discover and treat the cause of their pain. This book is part of that plan.

What you are about to read is not taught in the school systems...yet. We've been raised on the notion that health comes from the inside of a medicine cabinet, and that the cure is a pill, potion, puncture or powder, rather than we have an innate ability to heal. People often get frustrated treating the symptoms, rather than the cause of their pain.

I wrote this book to provide a set of steps - that anyone can go through - and identify what's going on and how to fix it.

Whether you are using this for general knowledge or a true "9 step process blueprint" - I hope this information helps reveal how truly awesome the human body is, and if given the correct environment, how it can work hard to make you pain free again.

To view my video series on top questions about pain, just scan this QR code:

Or visit my site: www.getridofmypainnow.com

Enjoy the book!

Dr. Jerry B. Dreessen DC, CCSP

DEDICATION

To all my patients who taught me the reality behind my instructions.

...AND THANKS

To my wife - for sharing her awesome editing skills

To Steve at www.stevebartlettphotography.com for his "eyes and talent"

To WhoIsYourWebguy.com for their expertise to help me spread the word regarding health.

To my dad who, after breaking his back in high school and was in a body cast his senior year, was told he'd never walk again without pain - was healed by a Doctor of Chiropractic. He decided to become a chiropractor - and is still living drug free. He passed his skill and knowledge to me, and is the reason I chose this Noble profession.

CHAPTER ONE

Introduction

INTRODUCTION

Susan was 29 and her birthday was coming up in a few months.

Was she ready to cross over the "line" and jump into the 30-something group? Here she was, happily married, raising 2 kids, and starting back to work. But something was different...

When she looked in the mirror, she knew her face and neck were puffier, the minor bags under her eyes were still manageable with makeup, but the overall puffiness, was persistent and the she just couldn't seem to lose the extra weight she'd put on since high school.

Trying to diet and workout were becoming more and more of a challenge. Was it the headaches or joint pain that was holding her back? The "head fog" and inability to focus seemed like it was never going to go away.

Staring in the mirror, soon to be 30, Susan was beginning to tear up. A mild depression was starting to form - a dark cloud almost visibly showing up above her head. A small, warm drop of moisture ran down her cheek she quickly wiped it off, smiled at herself in the mirror, and walked away, going through her mental checklist to make sure everything was taken care of before she left the house to go to work.

Once at work, she started off with the usual bang. Saying hi to co-workers, checking emails, putting out small fires. But then it hit again. The unfocused cloudiness. The start of depression. The yawning... the hunger. It was only 10:30 am, but for some reason, Susan always needed to have a snack of some kind between 10 and 11. She relied on a power bar, produced from her purse (purchased in bulk at the store), to aide her in coming back to the productive, working world.

A cup of coffee, some sugar, and a protein bar was just the trick to make it through to lunch.

She also had her usual bottle of NSAIDs to help with the 11:45 headache and neck pain she was about to experience from 90 minutes of powering through her "to do list" on the computer.

"Crap, not again" she said out loud. Her wrists were starting to burn. Not just a little bit, like usual, but a lot more. She found herself rubbing them and shaking them every 10 minutes. "This is only Tuesday" she said to herself. "I still have 3 more days to go!" She worked the next 90 minutes in agony.

To make up for lost time Susan cut her lunch short, making sure not to drink too much of her juice with her meal. Management didn't necessarily frown on frequent trips to the bathroom, but productivity reviews are how management considers your bonus, as well as promotions.

It was now getting close to 3:30, and her wrists were really on fire. Each keystroke felt like a small sting in her hand. Her neck was beginning to get sore. Her back was getting stiff. Regrettably, Susan was slowly coming to the realization she was not quite ready for a full week of work, and would need to take a sick day either tomorrow or Thursday, depending on how she felt in the morning.

Guilt, sadness and anger were all bouncing around in her head. Concentrating on her work was nearly impossible. Break time was still 45 minutes away, and her stack of paperwork was not getting any smaller. A sudden sense of overwhelming picked her up and slammed her down like a tourist caught off guard in the Hawaii surf.

Why was she so emotional? What was wrong with her? "Am I broken?" she thought to herself.

Sadly, the answer was...yes.

CHAPTER TWO

What's wrong with you?

What's wrong with you?

If Susan's story sounds a lot like yours - you are not alone. Thousands of women AND MEN begin to experience these problems as early as their mid 20's, become depressed or upset when they struggle to lose 5 to 10 pounds, only to find 5 to 10 pounds more weight gained. They get sick easier, their stomach and digestion go awry, muscle spasms and joint pain become more prevalent and they consume more and more pills, potions and powders to battle the "enemy within".

How is this possible? How do normal, healthy young people begin to feel old, tired, in pain and depressed?

My goal throughout this book, using Susan as an example, is to show you how easy it is to become a *Super Inflamed Person*, how to recognize inflammation, and how to begin eliminating inflammation from your life, step-by-step.

It may seem complex, but I am here to tell you - it's a simple solution.
This book is going to help you to:
1. Identify what's wrong.
2. Put together a proven program with resources to eliminate the problem.
3. Make sure it doesn't ever happen again.

The alarm started playing music. Once again, Susan slowly rose from her bed. Dragging her feet across the bedroom she stopped to make eye contact with the woman on the other side of the mirror again. Foggy-headed, she drifted off into a place of memories…

Susan grew up in a small town, and was very active in high school. She got above average grades and played on the volleyball team. She lived in a house with her mom, dad and older brother. Her mom stayed home and cooked the meals, dad worked, and occasionally they would go out to eat at the local restaurants in town.

She managed to make good enough grades to move on to a local college, and began a 2 year degree as a medical coder, someone who creates the billing for doctors and hospitals. It trained her for a good paying job with benefits in a short period of time. It was exactly what she was looking for.

College went fast, and studying took up most of her time. Meals were fast, and often happened out of sync with the rest of her family. Even though she stayed at home, she spent most of her time on campus.

A quick meal would consist of pizza and pop, or "instant whatever" that you just added hot water to or microwaved at the student center. Breads, cakes, doughnuts, coffee, creamer, hot dogs, mac and cheese, sandwich in a box, fast food burgers - you name it. Eating food on a tight budget often meant going cheap on quality too.

During her time in school, she made sure to get proper sleep, but found she needed caffeine to make it through classes. She would get headaches often, with all her reading and studying, and would rely on the cheapest headache medicine at the store. Sometimes she would take one or two more than recommended on the bottle or increase the frequency based on the severity of the headaches.

Tony was from the town across the valley. His best friend was working at the same place where Susan worked. One day Tony stopped by to see his buddy, and met Susan. It was an instant connection and after a year, they were engaged to be married. Tony worked nearby managing a retail outlet, and picking a home close by for a short commute to work for both of them was an easy task.

The next few years seemed like a blur to Susan. She was able to take maternity leave during the births of her now 6 and 8 year old sons. Both in school, she could easily work mornings, while her husband could pick them up from school and spend a few hours with them before she came home to take over. She often wondered where the time went, and immediately remembered her staring contest in the mirror earlier.

Snapping out of her daydream, she saw that it was nearly time to go home, and her pile of work was sitting there, looking back at her. Taking a day off just might mean coming in this weekend to catch up. With a sigh, Susan logged out, picked up her things and headed out into the parking lot for her 20 minute commute home. Everyone was jealous - most of them had at least 40 to 90 minutes of driving to grumble through. "See you tomorrow Susan", one of her co-workers yelled across the parking lot. "Okay" Susan replied, wanting to say "Maybe" or "I'm not so sure", but then that would require more time talking, and her head was still throbbing just a bit.

Once home, she realized there was no way she would be able to cook dinner. Time, hunger, supplies - all told her to go with canned and boxed stuff. Quick, easy, delicious - the kids fed, and laundry started, she sat down to watch news of the day followed by a dryer's worth of clothes to fold, and then bed.

When the morning came, Susan was even more bloated. Her head hurt twice as much as before. Her joints were painful and stiff, and the muscles in the back of her legs started to go into a painful spasm. She was so thankful Tony was up getting the kids fed and off to school. There was no way she could make it to work today, let alone out of bed. She made the call to work. As she stood in the mirror again, with the phone in her hand, she knew something needed to change. She didn't know exactly what needed changing, but she was determined by the end of the day to have enough answers to start her journey of getting better.

While she was searching online she found a book that talked about all the symptoms she was having, and how there was a natural way to begin feeling better, without medications or a litany of tests. The ebook laid out 9 basic steps to help her recover from her roller coaster of depression and pain. Immediately she started reading the book. It seemed like the pain, headaches, joint pain, muscle pain and spasms were very similar to hers. But it would be the following chapters, each one designed to eliminate her pain and symptoms in a very specific, ordered way that would not only educate her on what to do, but why she needed to do it, and then help her create a pattern of habits to help her stay out of pain forever.

CHAPTER THREE

9 steps to change your life forever

9 steps to change your life forever

Imagine being a person that has pain everyday of their life, with no clue how to fix it. Imagine finishing every sentence regarding an activity with *"...while I can"*

"I better go to the store and get groceries tonight, *...while I can"*

"I better go sign up for fall basketball one more time...*while I can"*

"I better go visit my grandkids, *...while I can"*

If that's you - then this book is perfect for you. Prepare to learn things about your body we should have been taught in 6th grade.

The easiest way is to magically crawl inside my head and glean the 32 years of knowledge from chiropractic college and the post grad classes I've taken, including microbiology, genetics, physiology, organic chemistry, anatomy & physiology (OK, you get the picture), to make processing these next chapters easy. But instead, I have the unique opportunity to share these concepts with you - concepts that will be brand new for some of you! What an honor for me.

You'll see that I've put together a list that outlines the steps, specifically, *in the correct order* that you should take to begin your journey to becoming pain free. If you come to a section that doesn't apply to you, feel free to skip it, or read it just for the information to help others. I suggest you read this entire ebook first, to get an understanding of what it is I am asking you to do. Then make sure you have the time and supplies needed to start immediately.

If any of you are currently seeing a doctor for any reason, the methods in this book need to be approved by him or her too.

I have had a few patients accidentally forget to mention medications to me, or history of surgeries, venous thrombi, CSF fluid leakage - you name it, and that one little piece of information can be enough to cause symptoms - that are treatable, but often caused me to scratch my head a little - and wonder what was happening until they remembered to tell me.

So - bottom line: Read this book first, involve your doctor, then follow these procedures.

CHAPTER FOUR

SECTION A: LAY DOWN THE FOUNDATION

STEP 1: Medications, Adverse Reactions, Substitutions

Susan's dad was a healthy man, so naturally it was a surprise to Susan to see the back of his hand all swollen up. "Is that a bee sting Dad?" She asked.

"Don't know what it is" he said. "Been to the doctor today and he can't figure it out either".

Susan began her search on the internet for "unknown swelling of the hand". She began going down the list of possible symptoms and way at the bottom of the list was a thing called pseudo gout.

"What the heck is that?" Susan's dad asked.

"It's like gout, only it shows up in other places" Susan answered.

"Can't be that, I'm on gout medication" replied her dad.

"What?" Susan said, "Why are you on gout medication?"

"Well, the doc thought it might be a good idea to take, since I was borderline for gout" he said.

"So you don't have gout, but you are taking the medication for it?" asked Susan.

"Yep" said her dad.

Susan looked up the gout medication and looked up the adverse reactions. She gasped. "Dad, did you know that this medication can cause auto-immune responses to hand joints if you've been taking it for a while?"

Susan's dad looked at her, and then his hand. He had been taking the medication for over 8 months. He thought the medication would help him stay healthy, not harm him. "I need to talk to my doctor ASAP" he said.

Soon after he met with his doctor, Susan's dad stopped taking the medication and his hand's swelling and tenderness went away.

Your homework:

Write down EVERY medication you take, including over-the-counter medications. Once you have done that, go to your computer and enter:

"[the name of the medication] adverse reactions" or

"[the name of the medication] adverse effects"

Write down what you find. Here are some real examples of what you will find when you research these drugs online:

EXAMPLE: "Aspirin adverse reactions"
Stop using this medication and call your doctor at once if you have any of these serious side effects:
- black, bloody, or tarry stools;
- coughing up blood or vomit that looks like coffee grounds;
- severe nausea, vomiting, or stomach pain;
- fever lasting longer than 3 days;
- swelling, or pain lasting longer than 10 days; or
- hearing problems, ringing in your ears.

Less serious side effects of aspirin may include:
- upset stomach, heartburn;
- drowsiness; or
- headache.

This is not a complete list of side effects and others may occur. Call your doctor for medical advice about side effects.

EXAMPLE: "Plavix adverse reactions"

Get emergency medical help if you have any of these **signs of an allergic reaction:** hives; difficulty breathing; swelling of your face, lips, tongue, or throat.

Stop using clopidogrel and call your doctor at once if you have any of these serious side effects:
- nosebleed or other bleeding that will not stop;
- bloody or tarry stools, blood in your urine;
- coughing up blood or vomit that looks like coffee grounds;
- chest pain or heavy feeling, pain spreading to the arm or shoulder, nausea, sweating, general ill feeling;
- sudden numbness or weakness, especially on one side of the body;
- sudden headache, confusion, problems with vision, speech, or balance;
- pale skin, weakness, fever, or jaundice (yellowing of the skin or eyes); or
- easy bruising, unusual bleeding (nose, mouth, vagina, or rectum), purple or red pinpoint spots under your skin.

Less serious side effects may include itching.

This is not a complete list of side effects and others may occur. Call your doctor for medical advice about side effects. You may report side effects to FDA at 1-800-FDA-1088.

EXAMPLE: "Oxycotin/Oxycodone adverse reactions"

WARNING: ABUSE POTENTIAL, LIFE-THREATENING RESPIRATORY DEPRESSION, and ACCIDENTAL EXPOSURE
Abuse Potential
OxyContin® contains oxycodone, an opioid agonist and Schedule II controlled substance with an abuse liability similar to other opioid agonists, legal or illicit [see WARNINGS AND PRECAUTIONS]. Assess each patient's risk for opioid abuse or addiction prior to prescribing OxyContin. The risk for opioid abuse is increased in patients with a personal or family history of substance abuse (including drug or alcohol abuse or addiction) or mental illness (e.g., major depressive disorder). Routinely monitor all patients receiving OxyContin for signs of misuse, abuse, and addiction during treatment [see Drug Abuse and Dependence].
Life-Threatening Respiratory Depression
Respiratory depression, including fatal cases, may occur with use of OxyContin, even when the drug has been used as recommended and not misused or abused [see WARNINGS AND PRECAUTIONS]. Proper dosing and titration are essential and OxyContin should be prescribed only by healthcare professionals who are knowledgeable in the use of potent opioids for the management of chronic pain. Monitor for respiratory depression, especially during initiation of OxyContin or following a dose increase. Instruct patients to swallow OxyContin tablets intact. Crushing, dissolving, or chewing the tablet can cause rapid release and absorption of a potentially fatal dose of oxycodone.
Accidental Exposure
Accidental ingestion of OxyContin, especially in children, can result in a fatal overdose of oxycodone [see WARNINGS AND PRECAUTIONS].

EXAMPLE: "Corticosteroid adverse reactions"

Treatments with corticosteroids for short duration (lower than one week), even at high doses, have few adverse effects.
The risk of adverse effects grows with treatment duration and increase in the dosage. Various disorders can be observed:

- Cushing syndrome characterized by lipid redistribution the face, edema and fluid retention (to be prevented by a diet low in sodium), hypokalemia, increase in blood pressure, aggravation of diabetes, atrophies, muscular weakness, fatigability, menstrual cycle disturbances, growth retardation in children.
- Adrenal insufficiency at withdrawal of the treatment, which occurs even in neonates when the mother was treated during pregnancy. The discontinuation of the treatment can also induce various symptoms: fever, myalgias, arthralgias.
- Bone disorders: development of osteoporosis which can be attenuated by the maintenance of exercise, calcium and vitamin D supplementation, a hormonal substitutive treatment after menopause or by a biphosphonate treatment. In addition, osteonecrosis of the femoral head can be

exceptionally observed.
- Neuropsychiatric disorders, various, difficult to envisage: nervousness, insomnia, depression, aggravation of epilepsy, increase in intracranial pressure in children.
- Ocular disorders after local and general administration: glaucoma, cataract.
- Hematologic modifications: increase of leukocytes and thrombocytes, decrease of T lymphocytes .
- Digestive disorders, ulcer with an atypical symptomatology and cause of bleedings, as well as pancreatic damages.
- Infections: increase in the risk of infections, bacterial (tuberculosis) or viral (chicken pox, herpes zoster herpes), or mycotic (candidiasis). The infection generally evolves with low noise, without fever. The vaccination of people treated by corticoids is disadvised, especially with live vaccines.
- Growth retardation: administered to children, long term administration to children can induce growth retardation requiring treatment with growth hormone.
- Exceptionally shock during their administration by intravenous route.

EXAMPLE: "Lipitor adverse reactions"
Get emergency medical help if you have any of these signs of an allergic reaction while taking atorvastatin (the active ingredient contained in Lipitor) hives; difficulty breathing; swelling of your face, lips, tongue, or throat.
Stop taking atorvastatin and call your doctor at once if you have any of these serious side effects:
- unexplained muscle pain, tenderness, or weakness;
- confusion, memory problems;
- fever, unusual tiredness, and dark colored urine;
- swelling, weight gain, urinating less than usual or not at all;
- increased thirst, increased urination, hunger, dry mouth, fruity breath odor, drowsiness, dry skin, blurred vision, weight loss; or
- nausea, upper stomach pain, itching, loss of appetite, dark urine, clay-colored stools, jaundice (yellowing of the skin or eyes).
Less serious side effects of atorvastatin may include:
- mild muscle pain;
- diarrhea; or
- mild nausea.
This is not a complete list of side effects and others may occur. Call your doctor for medical advice about side effects.

Aspirin can cause ringing in your ears, Lipitor will cause low back pain. As you can see, there are a lot of things to watch out for. Were you given this list when you took these drugs? How about your parents, spouse or kids? I believe it's OUR responsibility to know what we are putting in our bodies. If your healthcare provider did not sit down with you and read the adverse reactions of the medications you are taking, and you didn't leave their office with complete knowledge of what you took, it's time to get a new doctor.

Or even better yet - take the time to go on the internet and read up on your medications like I have shown above, and educate your doctor. You may be needlessly suffering back pain because of the statins you are on. A lot of medical doctors don't realize the pain can be eliminated just by replacing the medication with a natural product, CoQ10, or just switching to a different brand. Most people that are on statins are "borderline" and can drop their bad cholesterol just by eating half an avocado a day!

Please complete this step *first*.
The next 3 steps may not work so well for you if you don't know what meds you are taking, and their potential side effects. By the way - why are you putting that stuff in your body if you don't know what it can do to you? Do you really need to take it? Or are you doing it "just in case"? Did you know that the majority of pain meds have an adverse reaction of *causing more pain*?

It's your responsibility. Don't be a passive sheep when it comes to medications. Too many people rely on their doctor (or doctors) to know what they are taking. Doctors see hundred of patients. They don't always know what meds you are taking, or the adverse reactions, or cross medications.

Bottom line: "Know Thy Meds!"

STEP 1 NOTES:

1. What do you need to do:

2. Why do you need to do it:

3. How can you create a pattern of habits to help you know more about your medications?

(Jot down your notes here for quick reference - but feel free to get a journal if you need one)

CHAPTER FIVE

STEP 2: Hydration vs Super Salty

Some of my fondest memories are of science class in Jr. High. That's where I had my first exposure to physics, and chemical reactions. One experiment that stands out was called "Osmosis through a semi-permeable membrane". We put a starch solution or sugar solution in a thin membrane-like balloon, and suspended it from the top of a jar lid and placed it in it's opposite solution – starch in the sugar, sugar in the starch, and in plain water. Water would either go in or out of the membrane, swelling up or shriveling, based on how concentrated the solution inside balloon was vs the solution outside in the container.

What does that have to do with our bodies? Well, to put it in another way, if we drink a bunch of fluids high in sugar or salt, our bodies become super saturated with salts and sugars, and no longer operate under optimum conditions. Muscles, tissues, organs and blood can be thick with all the salts, sugars, and medications people ingest on a daily basis, leaving their bodies starving for the best source of hydration: _water_ (sorry, but ice in your scotch doesn't count as a full day's supply of water).

So, how much water DO we need?

Well, how much junk is in your system? Let's start with that. What happens to all those toxins and salts in your body? Well for most of us they get caught in the liver, and the spillover ends up in our joints, which ultimately causes… wait for it… _inflammation_! Got sore, stiff muscles and joints? Feel 10-15 years older than you are? Do you get painful locking cramps when you stretch or bend? I bet if you start drinking more water, in a week's time, you'll notice how much better you feel.

Does it have to be _water_? Can it be juice, coffee, tea…? Sure - but remember this: you don't wash a car with dirty water. Anything that is in the fluid you are drinking will just slow down the hydration and _detox_ process (more on detox in the next chapter). As if that's not enough, caffeine drinkers have twice the problem because caffeine is a _diuretic_, which also leaches fluid of their body and can leave them greatly dehydrated by the end of the day. If that happens to be YOU, my advice is to match one mug of water for every mug of coffee you drink to stay ahead of the game.

These are the things I say to my patients, and here's what I hear back from some of them: "I don't like the taste of water", "I have to go pee all the time if I do that", "I don't get to use the bathroom at work whenever I want to". So to that I say, imagine a pot of soup on the stove, on medium high. Now fast forward five or six hours and notice how thick it's become with all the water that's steamed away. That's your blood, liver and kidneys when you are not hydrated!

So how much water should you drink? That's a very debatable topic. Typically 8 - 8oz glasses of water per day was the norm, but even that is changing. The most recent recommendation is taking your body weight and dividing by 40 (Example: 200 lbs ÷ 40 = 5 glasses). You should definitely have fluids throughout the day, and based on your activity and climate, adjust accordingly. I don't know why, but somehow drinking water became the "cod liver oil" of our generation. Those that need it can't stand it, or aren't sure what to do to make sure they are getting enough.

In my practice, I encourage water haters to just add ONE glass of water a day for a week and then see how they feel. Usually after a week they have added a second glass and are beginning to feel less "puffy". It is because of the results they are feeling, they decide to stick with it. Eventually they begin to like the taste of water, and add more volume and more frequency. So don't worry about not liking it.

Can you drink too much water? Of course you can. Water will also dilute your electrolytes - especially if you are drinking a HUGE amount. Some of you may be aware of the woman who died from drinking too much water back in 2007 from a radio station contest to win a Nintendo wii. She was 28 years old and drank nearly 2 gallons of water in a 3 hour period of time. It was unfortunate that the DJ's didn't look into the toxicity issues, and inform the participants. But 2 gallons in 3 hours is a LOT of water. Your daily requirements is up to a HALF a gallon, and it's over a period of 8 to 10 hours.

So what do you do if you hate water? Flavor it with a lemon, or lime, drink it with ice, have it hot as tea. If you are NOT drinking ANY water and you are taking medications, or smoke - why aren't you doing yourself a favor to be healthy? It's not only YOUR body, but YOUR responsibility to keep the fluid levels at a normal amount.

Bottom Line: Divide your weight by 40 and drink at least that many glasses of water per day.

EXTRA CREDIT: Drink Purified Water, get a water filter, or find a local Artesian well and stock up (use glass jugs - not plastic)

STEP 2 NOTES:

1. What do you need to do:

2. Why do you need to do it:

3. How can you create a pattern of habits to help maintain your daily amount of water

(Jot down your notes here for quick reference - and add more details to your journal)

CHAPTER SIX

STEP 3: NOW It's Time To Detox

Once you have taken action and started STEPS 1 and 2, you are now ready for the next step: detoxification.

Can you do detox if you haven't done steps 1 and 2? Yes. But it won't be as effective, and you'll still need to do those steps along the way if you want long term anti-inflammation to happen. In physiology class, where we learned about the human body and how it functions, my professor used to joke about how we were just "one long modified tube", where food goes in one end, gets altered, and then comes out the other end.

That truly is a very basic concept, and we also need to talk about the absorption of nutrients, fluid filtration and solid filtration happening along the way. Certain types of foods that we eat may not go through the system completely. A very mild, sticky, gooey "sludge" can begin to adhere to the inside wall of our digestive tract (the small and large intestines) and cause lots of symptoms. Fatigue and headaches, back and joint pain can be caused from this "reputrification" - constantly trying to absorb decaying particles into our systems. Heavy metals, impurities and fatty foods, all begin to turn into a layer of poison that our body continues to absorb into our blood stream, with major symptoms and consequences.

So how does a person "detox"? The simple way to understand it, is to give your body certain foods that absorb toxins, and loosen the gooey layer that is stuck to the inside lining of your digestive tract. Usually a 3 – 5 day or 10 – 12 day detox program works the best. I have links to companies that have good detox products listed at the end of the book. Also, if you have around 40 minutes of extra time this week, I suggest you watch one of my YouTube videos of an in-house lecture I did on detox to get a little more in-depth education than the 9 Steps goes into.

Some advanced warning: there are some people who need to take their detox program really slowly, and often need to repeat it. Removing the goo can often release all of the toxins back into the blood supply, which is not a fun experience. Headaches, nausea, chills and fever can often accompany a detox -

which is OK. These types of reactions can be controlled by dilution of the products to reduce, or decrease the symptoms.

If you have never done a detoxification, and have a dining lifestyle that includes a lot of cheese, meat, sugar and flour - I highly recommend that you do not skip this step. The thick layer of "goo" you most likely have literally blocks the ability to absorb healthy nutrients. Inability to absorb healthy nutrients because of a toxic barrier will not help you eliminate inflammation from your body, and may cause a sudden increase in allergies - which is why NOW is the time to do this.

To prepare for a detox, my suggestion is to do a smaller timed version. Begin on a friday, and plan time off to rest saturday and sunday. If your workweek is different, plan accordingly. Sometimes you can feel a bit cold, so bundle up as well - even if it is 80 or 90 degrees outside. You'll also need to drink plenty of water, which is why I had you start that with STEP 2. If you've been following this in order, drinking up to 64 oz of water is a breeze, and should not be a barrier in the detox program. Again - make sure you check with your doctor before going on this program. You body may have been absorbing a smaller percentage of your medications due to this sludge layer. Once your remove this, you body may begin to absorb a higher dose from the same amount. Our concerns include adverse reactions due to medication, or genetic disorders that may suggest you attempt other versions of this detox program. Feel free to email me if you have any questions as well.

Bottom Line: Eliminate the Sludge with a Detox - feel better, focus better.

STEP 3 NOTES:

1. What do you need to do:

2. Why do you need to do it:

3. How can you create a pattern of habits to help decrease the need for a detox:

(Jot down your notes here for quick reference - and add more details to your journal)

CHAPTER SEVEN

STEP 4: Fish Oil - The Natural Anti-Inflammatory

While getting my Certification as an Auto Injury Specialist back in 1995, I sat in on a lecture by a well known Chiropractor. His studies were showing amazing results. Not only were injured people healing faster, but their pain and inflammation were going away faster. He also noticed that their brain functions were getting better too. His new drug? Fish Oil. You may know it as "cod liver oil" that your mom and dad took, or the "castor oil" kids took in the 50's and 60's. It turns out that the pharmaceutical companies also studied the special properties in fish oil and tried to create their own versions. Unfortunately their new drugs were released to the public under prescription by physician only and, with a very sad ending. *They killed a lot of people.* You may know them as Celebrex, Vioxx and Bextra. The studies also showed great news that by the 85th day of taking 2,000mg - 5,000mg of fish oil, the subjects no longer requested NSAIDS and preferred taking just the fish oil.

Since that initial lecture, I now have all my auto accident patients taking fish oil immediately, and it has helped them recover much faster, with less chronic pain as they get older. Just like in the study, they prefer fish oil over NSAIDS. They are much happier knowing that their digestive tract, liver and kidneys are no longer getting irritated and inflamed.

Did you know that the main nutrient in fish oil (DHA) is the same as our brains? Yep. Fish oil is brain food. Stroke victims, people with concussions or other head injuries or mental illness can all benefit from fish oil.

Did you ALSO know that fish oil can help make you skinny? Yep. Fish oil also breaks down arachadonic acid, which accumulates around the mid section of guys, and the hips of women, helping you reduce that spare tire, belly fat and saddle bags.

Anti-inflammatory, Brain Food, Weight Loss - Fish oil is literally a *Triple Rainbow* when it comes to health!

So, let's review: now that you have reduced unnecessary medications, increased your water intake and performed a detoxification program, you should begin to feel better. In fact, a LOT BETTER.

You may begin to notice less phlegm in your throat, or that your sinus passages are no longer clogged up. Food may taste better, your sleep may be a bit deeper and some of the pain and inflammation may be a notch or two less. Some people going into this program with their pain scale from 1 to 10 (10 being the highest) start as a 7 or 8, and are now down to a 4 or a 5. Big difference for such small changes in diet and lifestyle. But remember - the more toxic you are, the more susceptible to allergies and colds and inflammation you become. Your immune system has been under attack for years, if not your whole life. You are just beginning to see the light at the end of the tunnel, and your outlook on life can appear to be a bit brighter, especially since your eyes are clearing up!

Now is the perfect time to introduce to your system one of the oldest, natural anti-inflammatories around. Fish oil. Yep - Mom and Dad's spoonful of cod-liver oil back in the old days was for a good reason – HEALTH!

So why does fish oil work, and why do we recommend it? If you can follow along with me through some organic chemistry 201 terminologies, I think you will get the BIG picture.

Cox enzymes convert the omega-6 fatty acid arachidonic acid into the pro-inflammatory pain producer prostaglandin E2 (PGE2). So if there was a way to stop or inhibit the Cox enzymes (I, II or III), the creation of pain would be lowered or stopped.

Pharmaceutical Researchers came up with a few products to do that. NSAIDs aka "non-steroidal anti-inflammatory drugs" like aspirin, ibuprofen, etc blocked Cox I and Cox II and reduced pain, but because of the blocking of Cox I, they caused a lot of bleeding (16,500 bleeding deaths per year). So the search was on for just a Cox II inhibitor, and believe it or not, THREE were created and approved by the FDA (Bextra, Vioxx and Celebrex).

In 2004, all three were pulled from the market (all started in 1999) because it tripled or quadrupled the incidence of heart attacks or strokes via another product called LOX. Published accounts stated that Vioxx resulted in 56,000 heart attacks during the 5 year release.
SEE REFERENCE SECTION FOR MORE DETAILS

What were these drugs trying to do? Reduce pain and inflammation. They were also trying to copy the natural properties of OMEGA -3 Fish Oils.

The OMEGA 3 properties in fish oil reduce the production of inflammation by breaking down arachadonic acid at the source, leaving no buildup of COX I, II, III or the stroke inducing LOX

Bottom Line: 85 days of fish oil can stop the need for daily NSAIDS, builds brain cells, and reduces YOUR "bottom line" (pun intended).

STEP 4 NOTES:

1. What do you need to do:

2. Why do you need to do it:

3. How can you create a pattern of habits to help?

(Jot down your notes here for quick reference - and add more details to your journal)

CHAPTER EIGHT

SECTION B: BEGIN THE REPAIR PROCESS

STEP 5: Begin the Anti-Inflammatory Diet/leptin resistance diet

Section B is a pretty big step, and a bit of a change from Section A. In Section A we were all about eliminating those things that were part of your past that were causing inflammation. Sort of a "re-birth" to your system. That's really the toughest part. It's like having to clean your room, or the garage, or for some of you - completely moving out of your house and into a new one! That's a lot of cleaning!

Since we metaphorically have a "nice shiny clean room", we need to make sure we don't bring in anymore "dirt". And by that I mean things that we are allergic to, potential toxins, and a closer look at the big three: flour, corn and sugar.

Most of us have grown up eating breads, cakes, sweet things from the store, juices, etc. Unfortunately our bodies are kind of like a "bucket", and each food has its own shape and size bucket inside us of what it can tolerate over our lifetime. Imagine having a bucket for flour, a bucket for corn/high fructose corn syrup and a bucket for sugar. Once that bucket is full, we get inflamed. The longer we stay inflamed and eat that type of food, the longer it takes to introduce it back into our system (if ever) once we get it out of our system. It's almost as if the bucket gets smaller and fills up faster.

So the big take-home for this step is stay away from ingesting anything that may cause your body to become inflamed.

Did you know that inflammation is one of the main reasons you can't lose weight? You're body's innate intelligence has taken body fat and surrounded all your toxic poisons with it, to literally "insulate" you from danger. This is also why some people get really bad headaches and body pain while they are losing weight. As the fat cells get broken down into energy and water, the toxins get released back into the blood stream.

I know a lot of people who have given up on diets because of the amount of pain they were in. In fact, they would take more pain killers, which would cause the body to need more fat to surround the toxins from the pain killers! So usually the more toxins we have in our body, the more obese we can become, and the tougher it is to lose weight.

The fact that our body is inflamed and can't lose weight can mean that it is missing an important ingredient: Leptin. Leptin resistance is why people's metabolisms won't kick in. Dr. Leo Galland's book "The Fat Resistance Diet" is a great read for those of you may need this type of eating habit. The book is about eating non-inflammatory foods, and eating raw almonds to restore natural amounts of leptin back into your body.

Bottom Line: Don't fill your "toxic" bucket up once it is empty

STEP 5 NOTES:

1. What do you need to do:

2. Why do you need to do it:

3. How can you create a pattern of habits to help…

(Jot down your notes here for quick reference - and add more details to your journal)

CHAPTER NINE
STEP 6: Add the Nutrients That Repair - Antioxidants

Let's imagine a brick house on a street. The house has been around for a while, and is made of multiple colored bricks. All of a sudden, a big truck smashes right through the corner of the house. No one is hurt, but you have structural damage. Here's the question: do you rebuild the house with one color of brick, or do you use multiple color bricks? If you want to retain the value of the house, you need to do the latter.

You need to repair your body is the same way. Now that you've eliminated the sources of pain and inflammation, and you have hauled out the trash, it's time for some rejuvenation. Enter the antioxidants. These little gems go into the body and create the foundation of repair. The body will take these nutrients and begin to build all the things it is missing.

So what should you eat? Brace yourself: *Real food.*

Not just packaged-add-hot-water stuff you buy off the shelves food. Stuff I like to call "1st generation food" - if you go back one generation, it was the ground. Literally from the dirt or branch to your stomach.

What SHOULDN'T you eat? Processed food.

Bleached, processed, hydrolyzed, enriched, high-fructose corn syrup infused - you name it. You don't rebuild a brick house with marshmallows. Get the point?

What if you don't have time to eat right? Let me be frank here: MAKE THE TIME. Ever heard of the phrase "A bowl full of skinny tastes better than any dessert"? Plan a day each week to purchase your food. Cook it up and take it to lunch. Provide snacks that fill you up, but are good for you. Still impossible? I have included a few websites that have all you need in the references section. Wasn't that nice of me?

Some patients complain that it can be expensive, yet spend $800 or more per month on pain medications, or 20K - 50K on a surgery due to a broken internal organ or tumor of some sort. Some of them buy into the illusion that they will go out of this world with guns a blazin', riding a horse into the sunset, when the reality is - they will be crawling across the desert with the buzzards pecking away at them. So don't worry about spending money on nutrients that will heal you. It's better than pain medications that can kill you.

So here's the list of foods to eat that do heal you:

1. Vegetables- not over cooked with salt and butter all over them, raw or steamed when possible, or even juiced.

2. Fruits - not boiled an in a can with corn syrup - fresh. Dark red or purple like blueberries is full of anti-oxidants.

3. Meats - if you are inflamed, you need to stay away from red meat. White chicken breast is your best bet, along with white fish.

If you hate the list above, go look in the mirror right now and look at yourself. Look at your eyes, your chin, your belly, your skin - do you want to spend the rest of your life the way you are with joint pain, and 3 bottles of pain killers, or do you want to be free of all that? If you really want to break free of this struggle - and believe me I know *it is a struggle* - get a friend, share this book with them, and have them help you through it. We've been de-programmed in our thoughts to say "Yah, but..." , doubting our every move towards health. Curling up in front of the TV watching Netflix all day, eating chips and dip is not a daily exercise. C'mon - you can do it, I know you can. I've seen it happen - but you are the only one who can flip the switch. I can't help you win this battle if you are going to fight yourself to the death.

Bottom line: You are responsible for your health. Learn the right foods to eat, avoid the bad ones or face stagnation and sadness.

STEP 6 NOTES:

1. What do you need to do:

2. Why do you need to do it:

3. What ways can you create a pattern of habits to help

(Jot down your notes here for quick reference - and add more details to your journal)

CHAPTER TEN

SECTION C: DEEP TISSUE ADHESION AND GREASING ZIRCS

STEP 7: PNF, SMA, Pool Therapy, Walking and Chiropractic

1. Here's what PNF is and why you should do it:

Proprioceptive-Neuro-Fasciculation, or PNF is the body's ability to know where it is at any given time without and visual input. When you close your eyes and move your arm around in front of you, your sensors in your skin, joints and muscles are giving your brian feedback so you know where they are. Since the majority of adults don't have 30 minutes of recess everyday, we don't get a chance to really move around, and our sensors begin to fade. Stimulating these sensors again will help trigger a greater awareness of your body, better fluid exchanges in the joints, and will allow you to walk again without having to use your eyes to watch your feet.

Joint healing happens much faster with PNF. Low back injuries heal faster by sitting on a therapy ball and wiggling your hips and back for 20 – 30 minutes a day.

I find it interesting that Tai-chi is a form of PNF wrapped around meditation and prayer. It's like a human-motion rosary bead for you Catholics out there. Instead of going to the next bead and saying prayer, you hold a position or stretch with your body. What a great way to stay in shape – in multiple ways!

2. Here's what SMA is and what you should do to fix it

Somato-Motor-Amnesia, or SMA, is when your body and brain no longer connect in a normal way. For example, a person who is under a lot of stress may walk around with their shoulders so tight, that they are slightly elevated. Some might say they are close to being a pair of earrings. Ask the person to relax, and they say they are.

What has happened is the muscles have been so tight for so long, that the sensory input has "reset" itself so that the new position is the normal one. The brain doesn't know the old position ever existed.

Here's how to fix it (for example, the shoulder scenario): have the person sit down in a chair and raise their shoulders as high as they can. Gently push their shoulders down while they push up against you. This is not a contest - they should yield to your pressure. As their shoulders lower, you will actually be pushing them back down to the real "normal". Repeat this procedure 3 more times. Always go slowly.

As the person experiences this new change, the muscles and body reconnect, and the "amnesia" is gone. They can now lower their shoulders to the real normal position, and can tell the difference from where they were, to where they are now.

3. Ready to move on: *POOL THERAPY*

Can't walk? Here's why pool therapy is the best form of exercise for arthritis.

This isn't for swimmers. It can be, but for now I am talking to the group of people that can barely walk around the house, or are in fear of walking because if you fall - you may not be able to get up. Walking in a pool is the great equalizer. You can walk around the edge of the pool with your hand on the railing, and your buoyancy makes it very easy to walk and move those joints around. Toes, heels, ankles, knees, hips, sacrum, spine - they all get a workout with a safety net.

Again, don't overdo it the first couple of times. Three times in a week is good. Get a pool membership at you local pool and go with a friend if you wish.

4. Ready to move on: *WALKING*

One of the most common mistakes people make on the road to health is the path they take. Taking an incorrect path with good intentions translates into an invisible dead-end to a disaster.

What do I mean by that? Simple: people who don't detox properly, or without proper education will often get so nauseated, or have diarrhea, stomach cramps, flu and fever, that they abandon the process. They never give themselves the time necessary to detox properly, and since it is without education, they give up thinking they should never do that again.

The same goes with exercise. Some people will start a walking routing, walk for a full hour, and feel great – only to wake up in the morning completely stiff and sore. It can take them up to 10 days to get rid of that soreness. Want to avoid that? I thought so:

START WALKING: 10 min at 50%

If this is your very first time exercising, you need to do a "test" of what happens to your body. I tell my patients to go out the front door of their house and walk away from it for 5 minutes, going just fast enough as if you were getting up to answer the phone. In 5 minutes, turn around and come home. Drink a glass of water. Stretch your hamstring muscles. That's it - you are done for the day!

Now wait and see how you feel in the morning.

Some people take up to 3 days before any soreness comes in. Why are you sore? Mostly because the fat stored in your muscles is being broken down into energy and water, and your tendons and muscles are yanking on the bones and joints. If you take time to let these processes toughen up slowly for the first 2 weeks, you can jump ahead quickly, without injury.

Some other things to consider if walking is your exercise of choice:
1. New shoes with good arch supports.
2. Comfortable socks
3. Water Bottle
4. Pedometer

5. Ready to move on: *CHIROPRACTIC*

My highest recommendation. If your joints are locked up, or not moving, a Chiropractor is what you need. Gentle joint manipulation to get the fluids moving around again, and to begin the initial phases of healing. I have included a handout on how to choose a chiropractor in your area to give you a guide on how to find one. Chiropractors are doctors that study the spine and joints, along with the nervous system, muscle system and blood system. Using hands-on manipulation they begin to mobilize joints and tissues that were once frozen or painful. You may find out that a diagnosis of arthritis is only a symptomatic phase, not a permanent disease.

You can also begin massage therapy, palates, yoga, tai-chi - all of these things begin to get the "juices flowing" and push out toxins. Just remember to keep your water intake up and start exercising slowly. If it is the summer time and it is warm out, remember to add even more water to your daily portions. Dehydration will also cause inflammation.

Bottom line: Begin to move the stiff joints without risking further inflammation.

STEP 7 NOTES:

1. What do you need to do:

2. Why do you need to do it:

3. What ways can you create a pattern of habits to help

(Jot down your notes here for quick reference - and add more details to your journal)

CHAPTER ELEVEN

SECTION D: NOW IT'S TIME TO LOSE WEIGHT

STEP 8: Weight Loss Program Can Finally Begin

Wait a minute doc, I thought weight loss should happen first?

Yep. That's what a lot of people think, and they often start *and then stop* a weight loss program because of 3 things: Joint Pain, Nausea, and Headaches. After reading the information above, doesn't it make sense to get your body READY to lose weight?

Inflammation is the reason our bodies are puffy, and why the weight loss mechanisms won't work. I'll even bet that those of you who tried a few of these diets and didn't get results could go back now and try them again, and get great results.

Pain, stress and poison are three things that our body will surround with fat to "insulate" us. The more toxic we become, the heavier we can get. Taking pain pills adds to the toxicity, and the body is forced to retain water and fat to protect us from becoming too toxic, sometimes causing organ failure or even death.

Protein, carbs, essential oils, vitamins, nutrients and water. That's what all good diets have in them. Don't starve your body quickly, or you'll trigger another bout of inflammation, and lose your momentum.

Which diet should you choose? I think the best way to view it is to imagine this: A dieting lifestyle, without convenience stores or fast food. Imagine living on a very special farm with all the fresh ingredients that didn't need preservatives. You could go wander around the farm and get whatever you needed whenever you were hungry. Fresh water, dairy products, fruit, veggies, meat, fish, fowl. I have listed a handout, and a book that I recommend from two different sources for you to get more information on diets. There are indeed many, many diets out there, and you'll find the one that works with you the best, and gives you the results you need. But do it without inflammation slowing you down.

But avoid sugar. Sugar is a very magical "hunger hormone". If you eat anything with sugar in it, your body will crave more food. I've had it happen myself a few times. When I've been eating like I should, and I have a bite of a cookie, or cake, and less than 10 minutes later - BAM! I need to eat a lot of food, and I need to eat it NOW!

If you have ever been off of sugar for a few months, you know what I mean. If you don't know what I mean - just know that you should be prepared to possibly get hypnotized by this fiendishly wonderful tasty bad product. Did you know that sugar is actually the best sweetener out there? It is. except for it's one flaw: *A very high addiction rate*. And it is no fun trying to kick the addiction, *or* the Type II diabetes that can result from it.

Some people reading this are already borderline and on the fence. Somehow Type II diabetes is creeping into your life. Your medical doctor is getting you ready to live a life of insulin shots, and you've heard about losing limbs and going blind. Not a very happy ending - unless of course, you can change your lifestyle and the foods you eat, reduce stress and unnecessary medications, and help your body burn the fat and improve the insulin resistance factors in your body that is needed to give your pancreas a rest.

Got a sweet tooth? We find that some people that can't stop eating sweet things can have low chromium levels in their blood. You can easily find that out by getting a special blood draw from your chiropractor, osteopath, naturopath, or medical doctor.

Bottom line: You can't lose weight and keep it off if your body is inflamed.

STEP 8 NOTES:

1. What do you need to do:

2. Why do you need to do it:

3. What ways can you create a pattern of habits to help

(Jot down your notes here for quick reference - and add more details to your journal)

CHAPTER TWELVE

STEP 9: Rest, Sleep, Repair

How much sleep do you get a night?
4 hours, 6 hours, 8 hours?

Do you wake up at 4 am in pain and just can't get back to sleep?

Are you getting deep, restful, happy dream sleep? If not, your body cannot recharge its batteries, and your brain can't categorize the previous days data into its storage banks properly.
There is absolutely no way your body can repair itself without proper sleep. It can become a vicious cycle of no sleep, no repair, more inflammation, no sleep, no repair, more inflammation, no sleep, no repair, more inflammation, until your body finally gives up and you lose.

How much sleep do you need?
There have been many studies out there that suggest a minimum of 5 hrs, but if you need to repair joints and tissues, I recommend at least 7 to 8. If you are a teen you need more - especially if you are in school.

I also recommend that you should't do TOO MUCH resting. It can shut you down mentally if you think you can't go out for a walk, or get up to answer the phone. As you can tell, I am only talking about the extremes here, and based on what you've read so far, I think you get the picture.

How old is your bed? What are you sleeping on? What about your pillow?

Golden Rule To Sleeping: The best environment produces the best sleep. How old is your bed? I bet if you can't sleep, it's because your bed or pillow is no longer supporting you. I'd rather you invest in a good bed, than have to switch one out every 3 years. I tell my patients that it costs about $200 per year for a bed. In other words, a bed that costs $600 will last about 3 years (600 ÷ 200 = 3). Anything made of foam will break down. Anything with springs will break down.
My advice on beds: Get one that lasts, that has a removable latex foam top (about 3 ") and is adjustable firmness. I recommend the Sleep Number Bed

above all beds because it won't break down, and you can change out the foam pad every 2-3 years.

Pillows are the same. Don't use a pillow that allows your chin to touch your chest. Your neck has a natural arch to it and needs support. If you are on your side, your neck needs to be supported for that too. A firm to medium firm pillow works the best for 80% of the people. I recommend the Chiroflow water pillow to my patients with over a 90% success rate.

Something else you can try: Stretching. There are great books on yoga stretches - get one to familiarize yourself with the basics. I recommend stretching the back of your legs, spine, quads, arms and neck and shoulders to help take out any tension.

Another recommendation: Melatonin. When your body is stressed, it can't make enough of this to help you fall asleep. By taking melatonin, your body is given the proper "code" to begin falling asleep.

If you can't fall asleep, follow this set of rules:

Don't drink caffeine after 5pm and expect to fall asleep at bed time.
Don't watch TV in your bedroom.
Crack open a window and get some fresh air
Use clean sheets
Don't let the pets sleep on you
Get your spouse a snore guard
Wear earplugs
Read a good book
Don't watch the news just before bedtime
Don't eat anything 2 hours before bedtime

Bottom line: Change your pillow, bed and environment to get better sleep

STEP 9 NOTES:

1. What did you discover about you from reading this book, and taking notes?

2. Which Steps did you identify with most?

3. List the steps you now need to take on a calendar, and put that calendar on the refrigerator so you can see it everyday. Also have a small list of 5 words or phrases of what pain free means to you (smile more, walk more, take the stairs, more family time, gardening… etc)

(Jot down your notes here for quick reference - and add more details to your journal)

As Susan set the book down, a new sense of empowerment began to rise within her. Not only did she realize she didn't have to live in a world of pain and fogginess, but she also knew there was a REASON that she was that way, and that she could do something about it.

That day she went to the bookstore to buy a journal for keeping all her notes. She began her journey, chapter by chapter. She learned about all the medications her dad was taking, and even went in with him to talk to his doctor about the reactions of some of his medications, and what other alternatives there were.

As soon as she reduced her sugar intake, and increased her protein and water, her brain fog and mood swings changed. As she went through each chapter of the book again, taking notes, she saw for herself what was wrong and what to do about it. By the time she finished her detox and started taking fish oil, she could already see changes - her wrist pain was gone, she could focus on her work, and her home life wasn't about survival; she could actually participate in a happy way.
Her headaches were a thing of the past, and with regular adjustments from her chiropractor and work station changes, she could move, bend and twist without joint pain.

As she looked in the mirror, she thought back to how gray her skin had looked, how furrowed her eyebrows used to be. How sick she had become and didn't know it.

Susan felt like her life had been given back to her. She realized her body belonged to her, and it was her responsibility to take care of it. The book she read was indeed a set of instructions to better health, and she took the chance and followed it. Once her aches and pains disappeared, she began to lose the weight she gained from her two pregnancies. She felt happier, thinner and the spark that had left her eyes finally returned.

Just like Susan, you've probably felt some of these symptoms. Even though she is a fictional character, she is the embodiment of many people I have treated. There can be multiple problems happening to your body at one time, that are virtually undetectable at first, but once the body's natural defenses start to break down, symptoms begin to show.

Now that you are armed with the knowledge of reducing and eliminating your pain, and inflammation, I want you to use the tools I have given you to make these great changes happen.

What they didn't tell us in grade school is that WE are responsible for US. No one has authority over your health. Never give your health over to someone who can misdiagnose and incorrectly medicate you without you knowing what you are putting into your mouth and body. We were told never to take candy from strangers. By taking medication without needing it, stressing out in jobs that have no outlet for anxieties, and shopping for fast delicious processed foods, we break a lot of rules we would never allow our kids to break.

You are responsible for you.

Toxins and processed food goes in, inflammation, pain and fat result.

Now go out there and get your feel good back on.

–Dr. Jerry Dreessen DC, CCSP
(Send your emails to questions@getridofmypainnow.com)

***Please feel free to email me your list or journal notes. I am interested to see what results you come up with, and what goals you have set. Please give your permission if it is alright for me to "anonymously" post your results on a special section on my website.

CHAPTER THIRTEEN

PRODUCTS

PRODUCTS • VIDEOS • HANDOUTS

Here is a small list of links that I recommend for the 9 Steps.

*For those of you reading the printed version, you can access the hyperlinks by going to:

http://getridofmypainnow.com/printlinks

PRODUCTS- I have used these successfully in my clinic, as well as my personal use at home:

Greens First Website
Longevity Anti-Inflammatory Product website
Biogenesis food supplements (password: 4HEALTH)
Detox Products
UltraLean Health Weight Management Program Handbook
Dr. Jerry Mixons book on healthy food and dieting
Zrii Detox Products

VIDEO LINKS- Just the tip of the iceberg, and very informative:

Understanding Concussion and Brain Injuries
Preventing Workplace Pain
Interactive 3-D Spine

Weight loss seminar
Detox Seminar

Handouts
How To Find A Chiropractor In Your Hometown

For Further Reading
The Fat Resistance Diet

CHAPTER FOURTEEN

REFERENCES

REFERENCES

Here is a small list of references to help you research the most current information on the 9 steps I've outlined above. This is by no means a complete list, but it will get you pointed in the right direction...

Spine Pain and Omega-3 Essential Fatty Acids
Dan Murphy, DC
Cox enzymes (Cyclooxygenase, officially known as prostaglandin-endoperoxide synthase, or PTGS) convert the omega-6 fatty acid arachidonic acid into the pro-inflammatory pain producer prostaglandin E2 (PGE2).

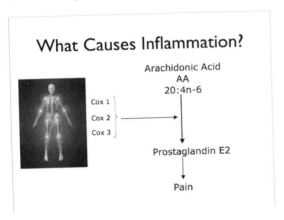

What Causes Inflammation?

Arachidonic Acid
AA
20:4n-6

Cox 1
Cox 2
Cox 3

Prostaglandin E2

Pain

Most cox-enzyme inhibiting pain drugs known as non-steroidal anti-inflammatory drugs (NSAIDs) inhibit both cox-1 and cox-2 enzymes. However, blocking the cox-1 enzyme resulted in significant bleeding problems. A study published in the New England Journal of Medicine in 1999 (1) noted that prescription NSAIDs for rheumatoid and degenerative arthritis alone conservatively accounted for a minimum of 16,500 fatal bleeding deaths per year in the US, which is the 15th leading cause of death in the US. It was thought that if a drug could be developed that blocked only the cox-2 enzyme, there would be fewer bleeding problems / deaths while maintaining significant pain reduction. Starting in 1999, the US Food and Drug Administration (FDA) approved three such cox-2 enzyme inhibitors, Bextra, Vioxx, and Celebrex.

On September 30, 2004, Merck, the maker of the cox-2 inhibiting drug Vioxx, pulled this product from the marketplace because it tripled or quadrupled the incidence of heart attacks and strokes. Bextra had already been pulled from the market for the same reason, and the FDA issued a "black box" warning (strongest possible warning against using the product without actually removing the drug from

2 the marketplace) against the drug Celebrex. Published accounts suggest that the

drug Vioxx resulted in 56,000 fatal heart attacks / strokes in the 5 years it was on the market (see reference #2 for review).

The scrutiny concerning the dangers of the cox-2 enzyme inhibiting drugs expanded to all NSAIDs, including those sold over-the-counter. An article published in 2005 notes (3):

More Pain Relievers Called Into Question
Study Stirs Concern About Heart Safety of Over-Counter Drugs
Associated Press April 19, 2005
By Marilynn Marchione

"With prescription drugs Vioxx and Bextra already pulled from the market, a study has raised disturbing questions about the heart safety of over-the-counter pain relievers such as Advil, Motrin and Aleve."

Those taking the "drugs for at least 6 months had twice the risk of dying of a heart attack, stroke or other heart-related problem."

The study was released at an American Association for Cancer Research conference in Anaheim.

"The findings add to the suspicion that the heart risk extends beyond the so-called COX-2 drugs – Bextra, Vioxx and Celebrex – to the larger family of medications known as non-steroidal anti-inflammatory drugs, or NSAIDs, which include naproxen, ibuprofen and virtually all other over- the-counter pain relievers."

"'To the best of our knowledge, these are the first data to support putting a [black] box warning on NSAIDs, not just COX-2s' said Dr. Andrew Dannenberg, a Cornell University scientist who helped do the study."

"The NSAID users were dying at twice the rate of the others from heart related problems."

"Risk was highest among ibuprofen users who were nearly three times more likely to die of cardiovascular disease than non NSAID users."

It is clear, that a non-drug approach to pain management is imperative. Dr. Joseph Maroon, neurosurgeon and specialist in degenerative spine disease at the University of Pittsburgh reported on such a non-drug alternative to the treatment of chronic spine pain on April 19th at the 73rd meeting of the American

Association of
3 Neurological Surgeons. A review of his research was published the following day,
and notes (4):
American Association of Neurological Surgeons:
High-Dose Omega-3 Oils used to Treat Non-Surgical Neck and Back Pain
Doctors Guide, April 20, 2005 By Cameron Johnston
"Investigators at the University of Pittsburgh have treated chronic pain patients with high doses of omega-3 fatty acids – the ingredient found in many cold-water fish species such as salmon."
"The researchers say their findings suggest that this could be the answer to the adverse effects seen with nonsteroidal anti-inflammatory drugs (NSAIDs), including cyclooxygenase (COX)-2 inhibitors, which have been associated with potentially catastrophic adverse effects."
Patients who took high doses of omega-3 oils were impressed enough with the outcomes that they chose to continue using the oils and forego the use of NSAIDs.
The 250 study patients suffered from chronic neck or back pain but were not surgical candidates, and they had been using daily doses of NSAIDs.
After 75 days of taking high doses of omega-3s, 59% had stopped taking prescription drugs for their pain.
"88% said they were pleased enough with the outcomes that they planned to continue using the fish oils."
"No significant adverse effects were reported."
This omega-3 research by Dr Maroon was published in the medical journal Surgical Neurology in April 2006. Comments from the abstract include (5):
Omega-3 fatty acids (fish oil) as an anti-inflammatory: an alternative to nonsteroidal anti-inflammatory drugs for discogenic pain
Department of Neurological Surgery, University of Pittsburgh Medical Center
The use of NSAIDs are associated with "extreme complications, including gastric ulcers, bleeding, myocardial infarction, and even deaths."
"An alternative treatment with fewer side effects that also reduces the inflammatory response and thereby reduces pain is believed to be omega-3 EFAs found in fish oil."
At an average of 75 days on fish oil, 59% discontinued taking their prescription NSAIDs for pain and 88% stated they would continue to take the fish oil.
"There were no significant side effects reported."
"Our results mirror other controlled studies that compared ibuprofen and omega-3 EFAs demonstrating equivalent effect in reducing arthritic pain."
"Omega-3 EFA fish oil supplements appear to be a safer alternative to NSAIDs for treatment of nonsurgical neck or back pain."
The ratios of the various omega-3 essential fatty acids is important (ALA/EPA/DHA plus GLA, etc.)
References

1) Wolfe MM, David R. Lichtenstein DR, Singh G; Gastrointestinal Toxicity of Nonsteroidal Anti-inflammatory Drugs; New England Journal of Medicine; Volume 340 Number 24; June 17, 1999; pp. 1888-1899.

. 2) Murphy D; Cox Inhibitors and the FDA; January 2005.

. 3) Marchione M; More Pain Relievers Called Into Question: Study Stirs Concern
About Heart Safety of Over-Counter Drugs; Associated Press; April 19, 2005.

4) Johnston C; American Association of Neurological Surgeons:
High-Dose Omega-3 Oils used to Treat Non-Surgical Neck and Back Pain; Doctors Guide, April 20, 2005.

5) Maroon JC, Bost JW; Omega-3 fatty acids (fish oil) as an anti-inflammatory: an alternative to nonsteroidal anti-inflammatory drugs for discogenic pain; April 2006;65(4); pp. 326-31.

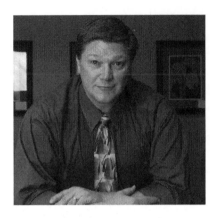

About the Author

Dr. Jerry Dreessen is a radio talk show host, speaker, author and nutritionist. He holds a degree as a Sports Injury Specialist, is a past team doctor for a Semi-Pro Football team, and is Board Eligible in Orthopedics. He is the Clinic Director and owner of Back To Action Chiropractic and Massage Center, in Mountlake Terrace, WA. His nutritional products and chiropractic procedures help patients decrease and eliminate chronic and acute pain associated with inflammation from injuries or lifestyles. His practice has been helping athletes, workers, cubicle jockeys, moms and dads and their families, live better lives by reducing and eliminating painful joints and muscles.

Made in the USA
San Bernardino, CA
24 May 2018